What you eat and drink can affect the way your medicines work. Use this guide to alert you to possible "food-drug interactions" and to help you learn what you can do to prevent them.

In this guide, a food-drug interaction is a change in how a medicine works caused by **food, caffeine, or alcohol**.

A food-drug interaction can:

- prevent a medicine from working the way it should
- cause a side effect from a medicine to get worse or better
- cause a new side effect

A medicine can also change the way your body uses a food. Any of these changes can be harmful.

This guide covers interactions between some common prescription and over-the-counter medicines and food, caffeine, and alcohol. These interactions come from medicine labels that FDA has approved. This guide uses the generic names of medicines, never brand names.

What else can affect how my medicines work?

Your age, weight, and sex; medical conditions; the dose of the medicine; other medicines; and vitamins, herbals, and other dietary supplements can affect how your medicines work. Every time you use a medicine, carefully follow the information on the label and directions from your doctor or pharmacist.

Does it matter if I take a medicine on a full or empty stomach?

Yes, with some medicines. Some medicines can work faster, slower, better, or worse when you take them on a full or empty stomach. On the other hand, some medicines will upset your stomach, and if there is food in your stomach, that can help reduce the upset. If you don't see directions on your medicine labels, ask your doctor or pharmacist if it is best to take your medicines on an empty stomach (one hour before eating, or two hours after eating),with food, or after a meal (full stomach).

Does it matter if I take my medicine with alcohol?

Yes, the way your medicine works can change when:

- you swallow your medicine with alcohol

- you drink alcohol after you've taken your medicine

- you take your medicine after you've had alcohol to drink

Alcohol can also add to the side effects caused by medicines. You should talk to your doctor about any alcohol you use or plan to use.

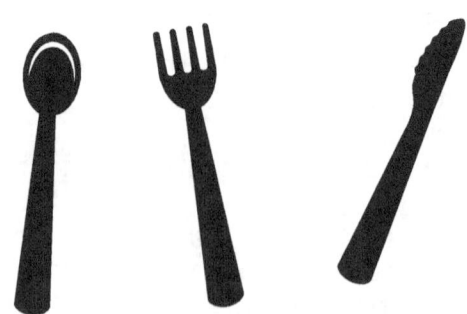

How do I know if caffeine is in my food or drinks?

Check the labels on your foods and drinks to see if they have caffeine. Some foods and drinks with caffeine are coffee, cola drinks, teas, chocolate, some high-energy drinks, and other soft drinks. For more about caffeine go to: www.fda.gov/downloads/UCM200805.pdf

Remember!

This guide should never take the place of the advice from your doctor, pharmacist, or other health care professionals. Always ask them if there are any problems you could have when you use your medicines with other medicines; with vitamins, herbals and other dietary supplements; or with food, caffeine, or alcohol.

What isn't in this guide?

This guide won't include every medicine and every type of medicine that's used to treat a medical condition. And just because a medicine is listed here, doesn't mean you should or shouldn't use it.

This guide only covers food-drug interactions with medicines you should swallow. It doesn't cover, for example, medicines that you put on the skin, inject through the skin, drop in your eyes and ears, or spray into your mouth.

This guide also doesn't cover drug-drug interactions, which are changes in the way your medicines work caused by other medicines. Prescription medicines can interact with each other or with over-the-counter medicines, and over-the-counter medicines can interact with each other.

This guide usually doesn't cover interactions between medicines and vitamins, herbals, and other dietary supplements.

Find out what other interactions and side effects you could have with the medicines you use so you can try to avoid or prevent them. If you have any questions, talk to your doctor or pharmacist. To find out more about how to use your medicines safely, visit the Web sites listed on the back panel of this guide.

How do I use this guide?

This guide arranges information by:

Medical conditions

Types of medicines used to treat the medical condition

Examples of active ingredients in medicines of this type

Interactions are listed by

Food, **Caffeine**, and **Alcohol**.

If you see...

- **A medical condition you have**

- **One of the types of medicines you use, or**

- One of your medicines used as an example here,

find out if **food**, **caffeine**, or **alcohol** might change the way your medicine works.

Allergies

Antihistamines

Antihistamines treat or relieve symptoms of colds and allergies, such as sneezing, runny nose, stuffy nose, and itchy eyes. They block the histamine your body releases when a substance (allergen) causes the symptoms of an allergic reaction. Some antihistamines you can buy over-the-counter and some you can buy only with a prescription from your doctor or other health care professional who can write a prescription. Some antihistamines can cause drowsiness.

Examples
> brompheniramine
> cetirizine
> chlorpheniramine
> clemastine
> desloratadine
> diphenhydramine
> fexofenadine
> levocetirizine
> triprolidine

Interactions

Alcohol: Avoid alcohol because it can add to any drowsiness caused by these medicines.

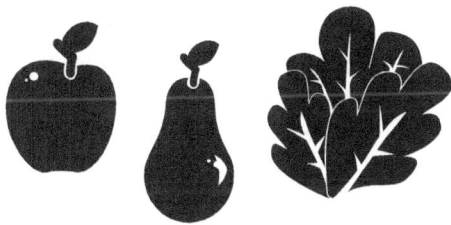

Arthritis, Pain, and Fever

Analgesics/Antipyretics (Pain relievers/Fever reducers)

Analgesics/antipyretics relieve mild to moderate pain and lower fever.

Example
acetaminophen

Acetaminophen relieves mild to moderate pain from headaches, muscle aches, toothaches, backaches, menstrual cramps, the common cold, pain of arthritis, and lowers fever.

Interactions

Alcohol: If you drink three or more alcoholic drinks every day, ask your doctor if you should use medicines with acetaminophen or other pain reliever/fever reducers. Acetaminophen can cause liver damage. The chance for severe liver damage is higher if you drink three or more alcoholic drinks every day.

Non-Steroidal Anti-Inflammatory Drugs (NSAIDs)

NSAIDs relieve pain, fever, and inflammation. Some NSAIDs you can buy over-the-counter and some you can buy only with a prescription. The over-the-counter NSAIDs give short term relief from minor aches and pains from headaches, muscle aches, toothaches, backaches, menstrual cramps, and minor aches and pain of arthritis. NSAIDs may be prescribed for conditions such as osteoarthritis (arthritis caused by the breakdown of the lining of the joints). NSAIDS can cause stomach bleeding.

Examples
aspirin
celecoxib
diclofenac
ibuprofen
ketoprofen
naproxen

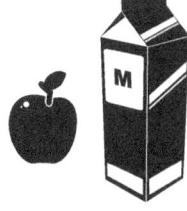

Interactions

Food: Take these medicines with food or milk if they upset your stomach.

Alcohol: If you drink three or more alcoholic drinks every day, ask your doctor if you should use medicines with NSAIDs or other pain relievers/ fever reducers. NSAIDs can cause stomach bleeding and the chance is higher if you drink three or more alcoholic drinks every day.

Narcotic Analgesics

Narcotic analgesics treat moderate to severe pain. Codeine can also help you cough less. Some of these medicines are mixed with other medicines that aren't narcotics, such as acetaminophen, aspirin, or cough syrups. You can only buy narcotic analgesics with a prescription. Follow your doctor's or pharmacist's advice carefully because these medicines can be habit forming and can cause serious side effects if not used correctly.

Examples
codeine + acetaminophen
hydrocodone + acetaminophen
meperidine
morphine
oxycodone + acetaminophen

Interactions

Alcohol: Don't drink alcohol while using narcotics. Alcohol can increase the chance of dangerous side effects, coma, or death.

Asthma

Bronchodilators

Bronchodilators treat and prevent breathing problems from bronchial asthma, chronic bronchitis, emphysema, and chronic obstructive pulmonary disease (COPD). These medicines relax and open the air passages to the lungs to relieve wheezing, shortness of breath, troubled breathing, and chest tightness.

Take these medicines only as directed. If your symptoms get worse or you need to take the medicine more often than usual, you should talk to your doctor right away.

Examples
albuterol
theophylline

Interactions

Food: Food can have different effects on different forms of theophylline (some forms are regular release, sustained release, and sprinkles). Check with your pharmacist to be sure you know which form of the medicine you use and if food can affect your medicine.

Follow directions for sprinkle forms of the medicine. You can swallow sprinkle capsules whole or open them and sprinkle them on soft foods, such as applesauce or pudding. Swallow the mixture without chewing, as soon as it is mixed. Follow with a full glass of cool water or juice.

Caffeine: Using bronchodilators with foods and drinks that have caffeine can increase the chance of side effects, such as excitability, nervousness, and rapid heart beat.

Alcohol: Avoid alcohol if you're using theophylline medicines because alcohol can increase the chance of side effects, such as nausea, vomiting, headache, and irritability.

Cardiovascular Disorders

These medicines prevent or treat disorders of the cardiovascular system, such as high blood pressure, angina (chest pain), irregular heart beat, heart failure, blood clots, and high cholesterol. Some types of medicines can treat many conditions. For example, beta blockers can treat high blood pressure, angina (chest pain), and irregular heart beats.

ACE Inhibitors (Angiotensin Converting Enzyme Inhibitors)

ACE inhibitors alone or with other medicines lower blood pressure or treat heart failure. They relax blood vessels so blood flows more smoothly and the heart can pump blood better.

Examples

captopril
enalapril
lisinopril
moexipril
quinapril
ramipril

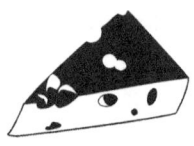

Interactions

Food: Take captopril and moexipril one hour before meals.

ACE inhibitors can increase the amount of potassium in your body. Too much potassium can be harmful and can cause an irregular heartbeat and heart palpitations (rapid heart beats). Avoid eating large amounts of foods high in potassium, such as bananas, oranges, green leafy vegetables, and salt substitutes that contain potassium. They can raise the level of potassium even higher. Tell your doctor if you are taking salt substitutes with potassium, potassium supplements, or diuretics (water pills) because these can add to the amount of potassium in your body.

Beta Blockers

Beta blockers can be used alone or with other medicines to treat high blood pressure. They are also used to prevent angina (chest pain) and treat heart attacks. They work by slowing the heart rate and relaxing the blood vessels so the heart doesn't have to work as hard to pump blood.

Don't suddenly stop taking a beta blocker without talking to your doctor. If you stop a beta blocker suddenly, you can get chest pain, an irregular heartbeat, or a heart attack. Your doctor might tell you to decrease your dose gradually.

Examples
carvedilol
metoprolol

Interactions

Food: Take carvedilol with food to decrease the chance it will lower your blood pressure too much. Take carvedilol extended release capsules in the morning with food; don't crush, chew, or divide the capsule. Take metoprolol with a meal or right after a meal.

Diuretics

Sometimes called "water pills," diuretics help remove water, sodium, and chloride from the body. Diuretics reduce sodium and the swelling and excess fluid caused by some medical problems such as heart or liver disease. Diuretics can also treat high blood pressure.

Examples
bumetanide
furosemide
hydrochlorothiazide

metolazone
triamterene
triamterene + hydrochlorothiazide

Interactions

Food: Take your diuretic with food if it upsets your stomach.

Some diuretics cause loss of the minerals potassium, calcium, and magnesium from the body.

Other diuretics, like triamterene (not with hydrochlorothiazide), lower the kidneys' ability to remove potassium, which can cause high levels of potassium in the blood stream (hyperkalemia). Too much potassium can be harmful and can cause an irregular or rapid beating of the heart. When you use diuretics that can increase potassium in your body, avoid eating large amounts of foods high in potassium, such as bananas, oranges, and green leafy vegetables, and salt substitutes that contain potassium. They can raise the level of potassium even higher. Tell your doctor if you are taking salt substitutes with potassium or potassium supplements because they can add to the amount of potassium in your body.

Glycosides

Glycosides treat heart failure and abnormal heart rhythms. They help control the heart rate and help the heart work better.

Example
digoxin

Food: Take digoxin one hour before or two hours after eating food. Try to take it at the same time(s) every day and carefully follow the label and directions from your doctor. Foods high in fiber may decrease the digoxin in your body, so take digoxin at least two hours before or two hours after eating foods high in fiber (such as bran).

Avoid taking digoxin with senna and St. John's wort since they may decrease the amount and action of digoxin in your body.

Avoid taking digoxin with black licorice (which contains the glycyrrhizin used in some candies, cakes and other sweets). Digoxin with glycyrrhizin can cause irregular heart beat and heart attack.

Lipid-Altering Agents (also called Statins)

Statins lower cholesterol by lowering the rate of production of LDL (low-density lipoproteins, or sometimes called "bad cholesterol"). Some of these medicines also lower triglycerides. Some statins can raise HDL-C (high-density lipoproteins, or sometimes called "good cholesterol"), and lower the chance of heart attack, stroke, or small strokes.

Examples
atorvastatin
fluvastatin
lovastatin

pravastatin
simvastatin
rosuvastatin

Interactions

Food: You can take most statins on a full or empty stomach. Some statins will work better if you take them with an evening meal. Don't drink more than one quart of grapefruit juice a day if you are taking atorvastatin, lovastatin, or simvastatin. Large amounts of grapefruit juice can raise the levels of those statins in your body and increase the chance of side effects. Some statins don't interact with grapefruit juice. Ask your doctor or pharmacist if you have any questions.

Alcohol: Avoid alcohol because it can increase the chance of liver damage.

Vasodilators-Nitrates

Nitrates prevent or treat chest pain (angina). They work by relaxing the blood vessels to the heart, which improves the blood and oxygen flow to the heart.

Examples
isosorbide dinitrate or mononitrate
nitroglycerin

Interactions

Food: You can take all forms of nitrates on a full or empty stomach.

Alcohol: Avoid alcohol. Alcohol may

add to the blood vessel-relaxing effect of nitrates and lead to a dangerously low blood pressure.

Vitamin K Agonists/ Anticoagulants

Anticoagulants are also called "blood thinners." They lower the chance of blood clots forming or growing larger in your blood or blood vessels. Anticoagulants are used to treat people with certain types of irregular heartbeat, people with prosthetic (replacement or mechanical) heart valves, and people who have had a heart attack. Anticoagulants also treat blood clots that have formed in the veins of the legs or lungs.

Example
warfarin

Interactions

Food: You can take warfarin on a full or empty stomach. Vitamin K in food can make the medicine less effective. Eat a normal balanced diet with a steady amount of leafy green vegetables, and talk to your doctor before making changes in your diet. Foods high in vitamin K include broccoli, cabbage, collard greens, spinach, kale, turnip greens, and brussel sprouts. Avoid cranberry juice or cranberry products while using anticoagulants because they can change the effects of warfarin. Many dietary supplements and vitamins can interact with anticoagulants and can reduce the benefit or increase the risk of warfarin. Avoid garlic, ginger, glucosamine, ginseng, and ginkgo because they can increase the chance of bleeding.

Alcohol: Tell your doctor and pharmacist if you drink alcohol or have problems with alcohol abuse. Avoid alcohol because it can affect your dose of warfarin.

Gastroesophageal Reflux Disease (GERD) and Ulcers

Proton Pump Inhibitors

Proton Pump Inhibitors (PPIs) work by decreasing the amount of acid made in the stomach. They treat conditions when the stomach produces too much acid. Some of these medicines you can buy over-the-counter to treat frequent heartburn, such as omeprazole and lansoprazole. Some of these medicines you can only buy with a prescription to treat conditions such as ulcers, gastroesophageal reflux disease, and to reduce the risk of stomach ulcers in people taking nonsteroidal anti-inflammatory drugs (NSAIDs). (See Arthritis, Pain and Fever-Nonsteroidal Anti-inflammatory Drugs above.) Proton pump inhibitors are also used along with antibiotics to stop infections in the stomach that cause ulcers.

Proton pump inhibitors come in different forms (such as delayed-release tablets, delayed-release disintegrating tablets, immediate release). Don't change your dose or stop using these without talking to your doctor first.

Examples

dexlansoprazole
esomeprazole
lansoprazole
omeprazole
pantoprazole
rabeprazole

Interactions

Food: You can take dexlansoprazole and pantoprazole on a full or empty stomach. Esomeprazole should be taken at least one hour before a meal. Lansoprazole and omeprazole should be taken before eating. Ask your doctor or pharmacist how you should take rabeprazole.

Tell your doctor if you cannot swallow delayed-release medicines whole because you shouldn't split, crush, or chew them. Some of these medicines can be mixed with food but you must carefully follow the label and directions from your doctor or pharmacist.

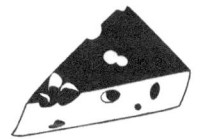

Hypothyroidism

Hypothyroidism is a condition where the thyroid gland doesn't produce enough thyroid hormone. Without this hormone, the body cannot function properly, so there is poor growth, slow speech, lack of energy, weight gain, hair loss, dry thick skin, and increased sensitivity to cold.

Thyroid Medicines

Thyroid medicines control hypothyroidism but they don't cure it. They reverse the symptoms of hypothyroidism. Thyroid medicine is also used to treat congenital hypothyroidism (cretinism), autoimmune hypothyroidism, other causes of hypothyroidism (such as after thyroid surgery), and goiter (enlarged thyroid gland). It may take several weeks before you notice a change in your symptoms. Don't stop taking the medicine without talking to your doctor.

Example
> levothyroxine

Interactions

Foods: Tell your doctor if you are allergic to any foods. Take levothyroxine once a day in the morning on an empty stomach, at least one-half hour to one hour before eating any food. Tell your doctor if you eat soybean flour (also found in soybean infant formula), cotton seed meal, walnuts, and dietary fiber; the dose of the medicine may need to be changed.

Infections

Be sure to finish all of your medicine for an infection, even if you are feeling better. All of the medicine is needed to kill the cause of infection. If you stop the medicine early, the infection may come back; the next time, the medicine may not work for the infection. Ask your doctor if you should drink more fluids than usual when you take medicine for an infection.

Antibacterials

Medicines known as antibiotics or antibacterials are used to treat infections caused by bacteria. None of these medicines will work for infections that are caused by viruses (such as colds and flu).

Quinolone Antibacterials

Examples
ciprofloxacin
levofloxacin
moxifloxacin

Interactions

Food: You can take ciprofloxacin and moxifloxacin on a full or empty stomach. Take levofloxacin *tablets* on a full or empty stomach. Take levofloxacin *oral solution* one hour before eating or two hours after eating.

Don't take ciprofloxacin with dairy products (like milk and yogurt) or calcium-fortified juices alone, but you can take ciprofloxacin with a meal that has these products in it.

Caffeine: Tell your doctor if you take foods or drinks with caffeine when you take ciprofloxacin, because caffeine may build up in your body.

Tetracycline Antibacterials

Examples
doxycycline
minocycline
tetracycline

Interactions

Food: Take these medicines one hour before a meal or two hours after a meal, with a full glass of water.

You can take tetracycline with food if it upsets your stomach, but avoid dairy products (such as milk, cheese, yogurt, ice cream) one hour before or two hours after. You can take minocycline and some forms of doxycycline with milk if the medicine upsets your stomach.

Oxazolidinone Antibacterials

Example
linezolid

Interactions

Food: Avoid large amounts of foods and drinks high in tyramine while using linezolid. High levels of tyramine can cause a sudden, dangerous increase in your blood pressure. Follow your doctor's directions very carefully.

Foods with Tyramine

Foods that are spoiled or not refrigerated, handled, or stored properly, and aged, pickled, fermented, or smoked foods may contain tyramine. Some of these are:

- cheeses, especially strong, aged, or processed cheese, such as American processed, cheddar, colby, blue, brie, mozzarella, and parmesan cheese; yogurt; sour cream (you can eat cream and cottage cheese)

- beef or chicken liver, dry sausage (including Genoa salami, hard salami, pepperoni, and Lebanon bologna), caviar, dried or pickled herring, anchovies, meat extracts, meat tenderizers and meats prepared with tenderizers

- avocados, bananas, canned figs, dried fruits (raisins, prunes), raspberries, overripe fruit, sauerkraut, soy beans and soy sauce, yeast extract (including brewer's yeast in large quantities)

- broad beans (fava)

- excessive amounts of chocolate

Caffeine: Many foods and drinks with caffeine also contain tyramine. Ask your doctor if you should avoid or limit caffeine.

Alcohol: Avoid alcohol while using linezolid. Many alcoholic drinks contain tyramine, including tap beer, red wine, sherry, and liqueurs. Tyramine can also be in alcohol-free and reduced alcohol beer.

Metronidazole Antibacterials

Example
metronidazole

Interactions

Alcohol: Don't drink alcohol while taking metronidazole and for at least one full day after finishing the medicine; together alcohol and metronidazole can cause nausea, stomach cramps, vomiting, flushing, and headaches.

Antifungals

Antifungals are medicines that treat or prevent fungal infections. Antifungals work by slowing or stopping the growth of fungi that cause infection.

Examples
fluconazole
itraconazole
posaconazole
voriconazole

griseofulvin
terbinafine

Interactions

Food: Itraconazole *capsules* will work better if you take it during or right after a full meal. Itraconazole *solution* should be taken on an empty stomach. Posaconazole will work better if you take it with a meal, within 20 minutes of eating a full meal, or with a liquid nutritional supplement. Don't mix voriconazole suspension with any other medicines, water, or any other liquid.

Griseofulvin works better when taken with fatty food.

You can take the rest of the antifungals listed here on a full or empty stomach.

Alcohol: Avoid alcohol while you are taking griseofulvin because griseofulvin can make the side effects of alcohol worse. For example, together they can cause the heart to beat faster and can cause flushing.

Antimycobacterials

Antimycobacterials treat infections caused by mycobacteria, a type of bacteria that causes tuberculosis (TB), and other kinds of infections.

Examples
ethambutol
isoniazid
rifampin
rifampin + isoniazid
rifampin + isoniazid + pyrazinamide

Interactions

Food: Ethambutol can be taken with or without food. Take the rest of these medicines one hour before a meal or two hours after a meal, with a full glass of water.

Avoid foods and drinks with tyramine and foods with histamine if you take isoniazid alone or combined with other antimycobacterials. High levels of tyramine can cause a sudden, dangerous increase in your blood pressure. Foods with histamine can cause headache, sweating, palpitations (rapid heart beats), flushing, and hypotension (low blood pressure). Follow your doctor's directions very carefully.

Foods that contain tyramine are listed on page 21, under **"Foods with Tyramine."**

Foods with histamine include skipjack, tuna, and other tropical fish.

Caffeine: Many foods and drinks with caffeine also contain tyramine. Ask your doctor if you should avoid or limit caffeine.

Alcohol: Avoid alcohol. Many alcoholic drinks contain tyramine, including tap beer, red wine, sherry, and liqueurs. Tyramine can also be in alcohol-free and reduced alcohol beer. If you drink alcohol every day while using isoniazid you may have an increased risk of isoniazid hepatitis.

Antiprotozoals

Antiprotozoals treat infections caused by certain protozoa (parasites that can live in your body and can cause diarrhea).

Examples
metronidazole
tinidazole

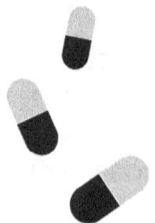

Alcohol: Together alcohol and these medicines can cause nausea, stomach cramps, vomiting, flushing, and headaches. Avoid drinking alcohol while taking metronidazole and for at least one full day after finishing the medicine. Avoid drinking alcohol while taking tinidazole and for three days after finishing the medicine.

Psychiatric Disorders

Depression, bipolar disorder, general anxiety disorder, social phobia, panic disorder, and schizophrenia are a few examples of common psychiatric (mental) disorders. Use the amount of medicine that your doctor tells you to use, even if you are feeling better. In some cases it can take several weeks before you see your symptoms get better. Don't stop these medicines until you talk to your doctor. You may need to stop your medicine gradually to avoid getting side effects. Some of these medicines can affect your thinking, judgment, or physical skills. Some may cause drowsiness and can affect how alert you are and how you respond. Don't do activities like operating machinery or driving a car, until you know how your medicine affects you.

Anti-Anxiety and Panic Disorder Medicines

Examples
alprazolam
clonazepam
diazepam
lorazepam

Interactions

Alcohol: Avoid alcohol. Alcohol can add to the side effects caused by these medicines, such as drowsiness.

Antidepressants

Antidepressants treat depression, general anxiety disorder, social phobia, obsessive-compulsive disorder, some eating disorders, and panic attacks. The medicines below work by increasing the amount of serotonin, a natural substance in the brain that helps maintain mental balance.

Never stop an antidepressant medicine without first talking to a doctor. You may need to stop your medicine gradually to avoid getting side effects.

Examples
citalopram
escitalopram
fluoxetine
paroxetine
sertraline

Interactions

Food: You can take these medicines on a full or empty stomach. Swallow paroxetine whole; don't chew or crush it.

Alcohol: Avoid alcohol. Alcohol can add to the side effects caused by these medicines, such as drowsiness.

Antidepressants-Monoamine Oxidase Inhibitors (MAOIs)

MAOIs treat depression in people who haven't been helped by other medicines. They work by increasing the amounts of certain natural substances that are needed for mental balance.

Examples
phenelzine
tranylcypromine

Interactions

Food: Avoid foods and drinks that contain tyramine when you use MAOIs. High levels of tyramine can cause a sudden, dangerous increase in your blood pressure. Follow your doctor's directions very carefully.

Foods that contain tyramine are listed on page 21, under **"Foods with Tyramine."**

Caffeine: Many foods and drinks with caffeine also contain tyramine. Ask your doctor if you should avoid or limit caffeine.

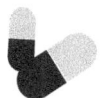

Alcohol: Don't drink alcohol while using these medicines. Many alcoholic drinks contain tyramine, including tap beer, red wine, sherry, and liqueurs. Tyramine also can be in alcohol-free and reduced alcohol beer. Alcohol also can add to the side effects caused by these medicines.

Antipsychotics

Antipsychotics treat the symptoms of schizophrenia and acute manic or mixed episodes from bipolar disorder. People with schizophrenia may believe things that are not real (delusions) or see, hear, feel, or smell things that are not real (hallucinations). They can also have disturbed or unusual thinking and strong or inappropriate emotions. These medicines work by changing the activity of certain natural substances in the brain.

Examples
aripiprazole
clozapine
olanzapine
quetiapine
risperidone
ziprasidone

Interactions

Food: Take ziprasidone capsules with food. You can take the rest of these medicines on a full or empty stomach.

Caffeine: Avoid caffeine when using clozapine because caffeine can increase the amount of medicine in your blood and cause side effects.

Alcohol: Avoid alcohol. Alcohol can add to the side effects caused by these medicines, such as drowsiness.

Sedatives and Hypnotics (Sleep Medicines)

Sedative and hypnotic medicines treat people who have problems falling asleep or staying asleep. They work by slowing activity in the brain to allow sleep. Some of these medicines you can buy over-the-counter and some you can only buy with a prescription.

Tell your doctor if you have ever abused or have been dependent on alcohol, prescription medicines, or street drugs before starting any sleep medicine. You could have a greater chance of becoming addicted to sleep medicines.

Examples
eszopiclone
zolpidem

Interactions

Food: To get to sleep faster, don't take these medicines with a meal or right after a meal.

Alcohol: Don't drink alcohol while using these medicines. Alcohol can add to the side effects caused by these medicines.

Bipolar Disorder Medicines

People with bipolar disorder experience mania (abnormally excited mood, racing thoughts, more talkative than usual, and decreased need for sleep) and depression at different times during their lives. Bipolar disorder medicines help people who have mood swings by helping to balance their moods.

Examples

carbamazepine
divalproex sodium
lamotrigine
lithium

Interactions

Food: Take divalproex with food if it upsets your stomach. Take lithium immediately after meal or with food or milk to avoid stomach upset. Lithium can cause you to lose sodium, so maintain a normal diet, including salt; drink plenty of fluids (eight to 12 glasses a day) while on the medicine.

Alcohol: Avoid alcohol. Alcohol can add to the side effects caused by these medicines, such as drowsiness.

Osteoporosis

Bisphosphonates (bone calcium phosphorus metabolism)

Bisphosphonates prevent and treat osteoporosis, a condition in which the bones become thin and weak and break easily. They work by preventing bone breakdown and increasing bone thickness.

Examples

alendronate sodium
alendronate sodium +
cholecalciferol
ibandronate sodium
risedronate sodium
risedronate sodium + calcium
carbonate

Food: These medicines work only when you take them on an empty stomach. Take the medicine first thing in the morning with a full glass (six to eight ounces) of plain water while you are sitting or standing up. Don't take with mineral water. Don't take antacids or any other medicine, food, drink, calcium, or any vitamins or other dietary supplements for at least 30 minutes after taking alendronate or risedronate, and for at least 60 minutes after taking ibandronate. Don't lie down for at least 30 minutes after taking alendronate or risedronate and for at least 60 minutes after taking ibandronate. Don't lie down until you eat your first food of the day.

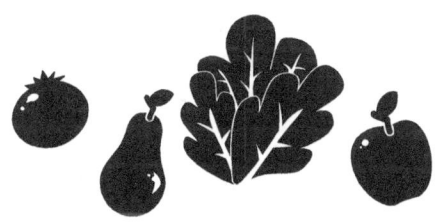

More About Using Medicines Safely

Read the label before you use any medicine.

Over-the-counter Medicines

Over-the-counter medicine has a label called **Drug Facts** on the medicine container or packaging. The label is there to help you choose the right medicine for you and your problem and use the medicine safely. Some over-the-counter medicines also come with a consumer information leaflet which gives more information.

Prescription Medicines

Medication Guide
(also called Med Guide):

This is one kind of information written for consumers about prescription medicines. The pharmacist must give you a Medication Guide each time you fill your prescription when there is one written for your medicine. Medication Guides are made for certain medicines that have serious risks. The information tells about the risks and how to avoid them. Read the information carefully before you use the medicine. If you have any questions, ask a doctor or pharmacist.

For more information on Medication Guides, visit: www.fda.gov/drugs

Patient Package Insert
(also called "PPI" or patient
information):

This is another kind of information
written for consumers about
prescription medicines. Your
pharmacist might give this to you
with your medicine. It gives you
information about the medicine and
how to use it. The pharmacist must
give you a PPI with birth control pills
or any medicine with estrogen.

Resources

http://www.fda.gov/usemedicinesafely
Consumer education on how to choose
and use medicine, from the FDA.

http://www.medlineplus.gov
Health information for consumers, from
the government's National Library of
Medicine (NLM)

http://dailymed.nlm.nih.gov
FDA-approved drug labeling written
for healthcare professionals, from the
government's National Institutes of
Health (NIH); sometimes this labeling
will also have a "Patient Package Insert"
or PPI or a "Medication Guide," written
for patients.

**http://www.accessdata.fda.gov/
scripts/cder/drugsatfda/index.cfm**
Drugs@FDA website with FDA-
approved labeling written for healthcare
professionals; sometimes this labeling
will also have a "Patient Package Insert"
or PPI, or a "Medication Guide," written
for patients. The site may have a "Drug

Safety Communication," or "Other Important Information from FDA," if there has been new information about the medicine that has not made it to the label yet.

http://www.fda.gov/drugs/ucm079489. htm

A personal medicine record can help you keep track of your prescription and over-the-counter medicines and vitamins, herbals, and other dietary supplements you use. If you keep a written record, it can make it easy to share this information with all your healthcare professionals—at office, clinic and hospital visits, and in emergencies.

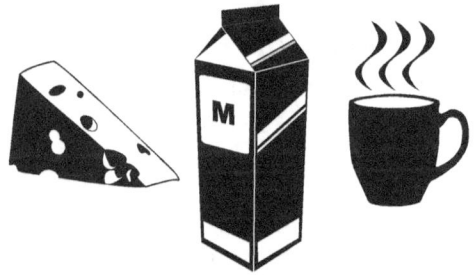